Irresistible Low Carb Recipes

Easy Recipes to Weight Reduction!

Robert Berry

Table-Of-Contents

Introduction

When it comes to losing weight, the nutritional options are endless. The diet industry rakes in $40 billion in the US alone each year. And yet, we - the people- keep getting bigger. That would seem to indicate that the majority of the diets being hawked out there aren't doing much more than making the bottom lines of some very large corporations fatter.

There are a few diets, however, that stand apart. They have stood the test of time, have millions of success stories and have scientific credibility. Sitting atop this list are Low Carb diets. The reason is simple . . .

Low carb makes sense and it *really* works.

For many, though, the thought of low carb conjures up images of deprivation and denial. After all, low carb means no cream donuts, no chocolate cookies and no soda! In this book, we will dismiss that notion once and for all. The low carb recipes presented within these pages are simply irresistible. Once you taste these exquisite delights, you'll hardly believe that food like this can actually be good for you.

The truth is that, not only are these recipes good for you, they will actually unlock the key to your new body.

We invite you to discover just how the low carb lifestyle can work for you.

Chapter 1: The Low Carb Solution

In 1960, 30-year-old Robert Atkins opened up a private medical practice in New York City. Over the course of that decade, Atkins developed a theory of wellness and weight control built around the controlled consumption of carbohydrates. He published a series of articles in the Journal of American Medical Association (JAMA) and, then, in 1972 he published his ideas in book form.

The *Dr Atkins Diet Revolution* took off. In the process it created a great deal of controversy among the medical community, with many doctors decrying the reduction of carbs as unhealthy, unsound and just plain silly. They also claimed that it was unsafe. All of this fed the media machine and made the diet more and more popular.

The updated *New Diet Revolution*, published in 1998, has been on the New York Times bestseller list for an amazing 6 years and has sold in excess of 5 million copies. Although Dr Atkins died in 2003, a massive industry has been built around his diet plan. To date, over 1 million people have successfully lost weight using the Atkins 4 Point Core Plan.

Eating low carb, though, doesn't mean that you have to follow the Atkins approach. The principles behind low carb dieting can be followed by anyone to achieve amazing results in every area of their life.

Low carb dieting can allow you to achieve . . .

> ➤ Rapid weight loss - up to 15 lbs. in 2 weeks
> ➤ Enhanced triglyceride levels - they boost energy levels and have a myriad of anti-aging benefits
> ➤ Increased HDL cholesterol levels - HDL (the good cholesterol) cruise the bloodstream, removing LDL (bad)

cholesterol, thus lowering a major risk factor for heart disease
- ➤ Improved insulin sensitivity - this allows more nutrients to get into the body's cells to build, fuel and repair muscle cells
- ➤ Decreased blood pressure - this reduces your chances of suffering cardiovascular disease and enhances overall health and well being
- ➤ Lower blood insulin levels - Insulin is a fat storing hormone, so it makes sense to get the amount of it in your body as low as you can
- ➤ Increased energy
- ➤ Reduced cravings for sweet foods
- ➤ Enhanced mental functioning - better concentration and improved mood

In addition to the above, many people have reported the following benefits of going low carb:
- ➤ Reduced joint and muscle pain
- ➤ Fewer headaches
- ➤ PMS improvement
- ➤ Improved gastrointestinal functioning

One of the first things you'll notice when you switch to low carb is that you are no longer feeling hungry every few hours. As a result you'll be eating far fewer calories each day.

The fat will melt off your body as a result of going low carb. But not only that . . . low carb dieting does a fantastic job of attacking the stubborn visceral fat that sits around the abdominal cavity. It also has a tendency to collect around your organs. This fat loss will not only make you look a whole lot better, it will also dramatically lower your risk of heart disease and type two diabetes.

Chapter 2: Low Carb Basics

What is a Low Carb Diet?

Low carb diets are designed to speed the metabolism and enhance fat loss by eating foods that are high in protein while simultaneously limiting the intake of high carbohydrate foods, which raise the body's blood sugar levels. The basis of the diet is the state of ketosis. Ketosis occurs when the body's carbohydrate intake is measurably reduced and the body needs to turn to its secondary energy reserve in order to fuel the body. That secondary reserve is stored fat. When we consume a high carbohydrate meal, we increase the body's production of insulin, a hormone that causes cells to absorb glucose from the blood. Insulin actually stops the body from using fat as a source of energy because it slows down the release of glucagon. At the same time it facilitates the conversion of consumed fat into triglycerides, which are stored as body fat.

A low carb diet is one in which you restrict your consumption of sugary and starchy carbohydrates. Your major sources of food are protein, fat, and fibrous carbs such as leafy vegetables that are grown above the ground. Those that grow below the ground, such as potatoes, beets and carrots are too high in sugar, and are, therefore, limited. There are a huge variety of low carb diets out there, the most popular of which is the Atkins diet. Each diet will have it's own restrictions on how many carbs you can consume.

Carbohydrates are found naturally in many plant-based foods. Plant based carbs are complex and fibrous. Carbohydrates that are found in milk and fruits are not as complex. Simple carbohydrates can be added to processed foods to add flavor and taste. The added carbs are in the form of sugar or flour.

Glucose is your body's primary energy source. When you eat or drink carbohydrates, like sugars, grains, starchy vegetables and high-glycemic fruits and dairy products, they are broken down in your body, and glucose is formed and released into your bloodstream. Insulin is released by the pancreas and helps to regulate the concentration of glucose in the blood.

Insulin is a hormone. It allows your body to use glucose (sugar) for energy. Insulin is made by the pancreas and it is what helps your body to use the glucose from the carbohydrates found in the foods you eat to either create energy or to store the glucose for use in the near future. Insulin helps to control your blood sugar, keeping it from getting too high or too low.

When you consume carbohydrates, they are broken down into glucose, which is a simple sugar. The glucose is then transported through your bloodstream out to the cells, where it is converted into energy. The amount of glucose in the bloodstream is very tightly regulated by insulin and other hormones. Insulin is continually being released in small amounts by the pancreas.

When the amount of glucose in the bloodstream rises to a certain level, the pancreas will release more insulin to force more glucose into the cells. This causes the blood glucose levels to drop. To avoid hypoglycemia (low blood sugar), signals are sent to inform the body of the need to eat, and some of the glucose stored in the liver is released. The liver also signals the body to lower the amount of insulin being released. Your body's main objective is to keep everything in balance: to keep your blood sugar at a stable level with the right amount of insulin and to provide the cells with the energy they need to perform their work.

One job of insulin is to stop fat burning and enhance fat storage. So, if insulin is the hormone that controls fat storage and fat metabolism, then by stopping our bodies producing insulin, we've got the answer to fat loss. The primary secreter of insulin is dietary carbohydrate. So, by cutting out the sugars and starches, your body won't be using producing extra insulin and it will be burning fat for energy.

How Carbs are Measured

Macronutrients are nutrients that supply our bodies with energy. There are three macronutrients:

- ✓ Carbohydrates
- ✓ Proteins
- ✓ Fats

When measuring food, the first important marker is to analyze their macronutrient breakdown. Nearly all foods will contain all three of the macronutrients. On a low carb diet you will be concentrating on foods that have a low percentage of carbs (less than 20%) and a higher percentage of fats and proteins.

Carbohydrates come as two distinct types. They are variously known as sugars or simple carbs and starches or complex carbs. The most abundant simple carbs are glucose, fructose and galactose. Each of these contains a single unit of sugar. By combining these simple sugars, new types of sugars can be made as follows . . .

Glucose + Fructose = Sucrose

Glucose + Galactose = Lactose (milk sugar)

Starches are made up of long chains of glucose. When we eat starches, however, they break down into individual glucose units. Most of the carbohydrates in such foods as potatoes, bread, pasta, cereals and rice are starches. Green leafy vegetables contain very small amounts of carbs, either as starches or sugars. They are, however, very high in fiber.

Fibrous Carbs can help burn fat: because fibrous carbs take more time to chew and swallow, fill up your stomach by adding bulk to your meal, slow down gastric emptying and decrease appetite stimulating hormones, they are a smart choice for those wishing to lose body fat. Another great positive is that fibrous carbs are very low in calories. That means that you can eat as many green vegetables as you want, without overdosing on calories.

A calorie is simply a measure of heat energy. Because food releases energy as it burns inside the body, the more calories a food contains, the more energy it will release. Body-fat is stored energy, much like a reserve gas tank for your car. Each pound of fat contains 3,500 calories. Each of the three macronutrients – carbs, protein and fat – contain specific amounts of calories. Carbohydrates and protein contain 4 calories per gram, while fat contains 9 calories per gram.

When calculating how many calories of carbs you will be eating per day, you simply multiply the total weight of the carbs you are eating over the course of the day by 4.

So, if you were to consume 100 grams of carb calories per day, then you would be eating 400 calories of carbohydrate per day.

How Many Carbs For Weight Loss

The simple question of how many carbs to eat each day is not an easy one to answer. That's because everyone's different and we all process and tolerate carbohydrates at different rates. The ideal carb intake for each individual depends on a number of factors including . . .

✓ Age
✓ Body composition
✓ Gender
✓ Level of activity
✓ Metabolic health

If you are very active physically you will be able to consume more carbs than a sedentary person. This is especially so if you are carrying a large amount of muscle mass.

The following guidelines, however, will work for 90% of people.

100-150 Grams Per Day

If you are already relatively lean, not carrying an appreciable amount of body fat and are primarily concerned with maintaining your health and your weight, then keeping your levels between 100 and 150 grams per day is ideal for you.

On this carb count you can eat as many vegetables as you care to. In addition, you can have a few small pieces of fruit and a small number of starchy carbs (potatoes, rice and oats).

50-100 Grams Per Day

If you have a moderate amount of fat to lose, you will want to ingest between 50 and 100 grams of carbs per day. That equates to a few vegetables, no more than two pieces of fruit and very limited starchy carbs.

20-50 Grams Per Day

If you want to kick your fat burn into high gear, then you need to restrict your carbs to below 50 grams per day. Doing so will put your body into a state of ketosis, forcing it to turn to your fat stores to supply the energy that your body needs.

Even though this is a low carb diet, it is not a no carb diet. You can and should still eat plenty of low carb vegetables such as lettuce, spinach, kale, bok choy, cabbage, mushrooms and asparagus.

Learning the Food Groups

In order to help people make healthy food choices, the US Department of Agriculture introduced the five food groups back in 1916. Although our knowledge of nutrition has grown in leaps and bounds over the last century, the five food groups can still guide us toward smart nutritional choices.

The Five Food Groups are . . .

Fruits

Fruits are crammed full of health giving nutrients, including antioxidants. Some of them, however, are also packed with sugar. On a low carb diet you should eat a maximum of three pieces of fruit per day. If attempting to keep carbs below 50 grams, fruit will be on the no-go list.

Vegetables

On a low carb diet, you will consume more of this food group than any other. The vegetables you will focus on, however, will be leafy vegetables, as opposed to the starchy vegetables that typically grow under the ground and are full of starch. Make sure that you get a variety of colors in your carbs. This will provide you with much needed phytonutrients and antioxidants.

Grains

Grains will be very limited on a low carb diet. Those that will make it through will be whole and intact, such as brown rice or barley. Stay well away from such refined grains as white rice or flour.

Protein Foods

A low carb diet typically means that you will be eating a sizeable amount of protein. Protein will keep your body in an anabolic state, allowing you to preserve your muscle mass while melting away the fat. According to the national Academy of Sciences, protein should comprise about 35% of total macronutrient content.

Dairy

Many dairy products contain lactose, which is a form of sugar. For this reason, you should limit your intake of dairy while on a low carb diet. However, such foods as cheese, cottage cheese and some types of yogurt will provide you with the goodness of dairy (protein, calcium) without the sugar content.

Chapter 3: Carb Counting Made Easy

Knowing just how many carbs are entering your body is important if you are to succeed on a low carb diet. Carbs, especially in the form of starch and sugar, are everywhere. Unless you keep on top of what you are consuming, your numbers can easily creep up. An excellent way to measure the number of carbs that you are consuming is with the *carbohydrate factor method.*

With the carbohydrate factor method, you multiply the raw weight of a food by the percentage of the weight of that food that is carbohydrate.

As an example the average banana weighs 120 grams and contains 18% protein. The calculation, then, would be as follows . .
.

120 x .18 = 21.6 grams of carbohydrate

Getting into the habit of measuring your foods on a pair of bathroom scales will allow you to accurately keep tabs on how many carbs are going into your system. But how do you find out what the percentage of carbs is for a given food? The simplest way is to consult the nutritional facts panel on the food packaging.

Let's consider the example of a box of Rice Crispies. If you take a look at the nutritional facts panel, you'll see that a single serving of Rice Crispies is one and a quarter cups or 33 grams. That single serving has 29 grams of carbohydrate in it. Now you are able to calculate the carb factor percentage as follows . . .

29 / 33 = .88 = 88%

We now know that 88% of a serving of Rice Crispies is carbohydrate. To work out how many carbs you're about to consume you would weigh your portion and multiply it by a factor of 0.88. Of course, if you were adding milk and a piece of chopped up fruit to the bowl of cereal, you would work out their individual factors and then add tem to that for Rice Crispies.

What about foods that don't come with nutritional labels, like fruit and vegetables? Simply check this site to find a ready-made list of carbohydrate factors (http://static.diabetesselfmanagement.com/pdfs/pdf_2074.pdf)

Counting Carbs and Fiber

Fiber is your friend. It will help to slow the rate at which the body breaks down carbs, thereby assisting in the management of blood sugar levels. Fiber also lowers your risk of heart disease, stroke, and it is extremely filling. This means that you'll feel fuller on fewer calories, a great bonus when you are trying to manage your appetite.

Because of the many benefits of taking fiber on board as part of a low carb diet, the fiber in your food will actually cancel out some of the carbs that you have eaten. Because fiber does not affect your blood sugar levels or your body fat percentage, you do not have to count carbs from fiber as part of your daily total.

To work out your net carbs (that is, your fiber free carb amount), subtract the fiber carbs from the total carbs. Here's an example . . .

A banana contains 24 grams of carbs. 3 of those grams are from fiber. The number of grams that will count toward your daily total will be 21 grams (24 – 3).

High Carb Foods

Refined sugar products such as white sugar, candy, sweets and soft drinks, are the biggest culprit in the obesity epidemic that is plaguing the Western world. Added sugar provides absolutely zero essential nutrient quality. As such they are known as empty calories. Sugar is also high in fructose, which can only be broken down by the liver. Too much of it can put overdue stress on your liver, forcing it to turn the fructose into fat and causing fatty liver. Sugar can also cause insulin resistance, which can in turn open the road to diabetes. There is also considerable evidence that too much sugar can contribute to cancer. Sugar, because of its ability to release dopamine in the brain, is highly addictive. And to top it off, sugar will make you teeth rotten.

A Dozen Processed Foods to Ditch Today

- ➢ Fried Foods (chicken, chips, onion rings)
- ➢ Biscuits
- ➢ Crackers
- ➢ Pies
- ➢ Doughnuts
- ➢ Margarine
- ➢ Tortilla Chips
- ➢ Refined Vegetable Oils
- ➢ Soft Drinks
- ➢ White Bread

➤ Pasta
➤ Bagels

Carb Counting When Eating Out

Eating out is one of the great pleasures of life. Eating low carb doesn't mean that you have to deny yourself of that pleasure. It simply requires you to do a little forward planning.

You should know before you leave home how many grams of carbs you are allowed to eat with your restaurant meal. Then it's simply a matter of estimating how many carbs are in the meal that is put in front of you. Follow this simple guide to be able to do just that . . .

Get to know how many grams of carbs are in everyday foods that you are likely to eat. Before long, you'll know these numbers automatically. If you're not there yet, you can download some amazing apps right to your phone and find out the complete nutritional breakdown of any food instantly.

Take a look at the food on the plate, or listed on the menu, and work out the total carbs. Many restaurants publish their menus on their websites, and even do the carb count for you, so all you have to do is consult their site to see if your desired meal fits within your carb range for that meal.

If the carb count of the meal you want is too high, don't be shy to ask your waiter for a low carb substitute.

Low Carb Restaurant Guide

To make it even easier to stay on track when eating out, here are our preferred selections when eating away from home.

Burger King

Whopper Burger
Grilled chicken sandwich
Veggie burger

ALL WITHOUT THE BUN!

KFC

Roasted chicken caesar salad (no croutons)
Roasted chicken salad
Chicken wings

McDonald's

Cheeseburger
Hamburger

ALL WITHOUT THE BUN!

Grilled chicken salad
Scrambled egg and sausage patty (no bun)

Subway

Any sub – order it as a salad!

Italian Restaurants

Prosciutto with melon or asparagus
Parmigiano Reggiano
Antipasto
Caponato
Unbreaded meat, fish and poultry entrees

Greek Restaurants

Tzatziki
Taramsalata
Avgolemono soup
Roasted, skewered, or grilled lamb, beef, pork and chicken

Mexican Restaurants

Salsa (no added sugar)
Guacamole with jicama strips
Grilled chicken wings
Sopa de Albondigas
Naked fajitas
Grilled chicken or fish

French Restaurants

French onion soup
Coquilles St Jacques
Steak au Poivre
Veal Marengo
Boeuf Bourguignon
Duck a'l'Orange

Chinese Restaurants

Egg-drop soup (no cornflour)
Steamed beef with Chinese mushrooms
Stir-fried chicken with garlic
Moo Shoo Pork

Extra Considerations When Eating Out

1) Don't believe the menu - just because an item is marked as 'low 'carb', doesn't mean that you shouldn't check the ingredients for yourself.
2) Control your portions – If there is too much on the plate, shovel some of it onto a side plate – and then leave it alone.
3) Ask for the salad to be served on a side dish. If you order dressing, make sure it has an oil and vinegar base.
4) Don't be tempted to make impulse eating decisions – exercise your self-discipline!

Low Carb Snacks

Snacking is often what unravels a diet. In between scheduled meals times you drift toward the no go foods, simply because they are there and you are famished. On a low carb diet, snacking is actually encouraged, provided, of course, the foods that you are eating are comprised of protein and fat. The right snack will keep your energy levels stable and prevent you from getting jittery. It will also keep your body in positive nitrogen balance so you can maintain an anabolic state.

You don't want your snack food to contain more than three grams of carbohydrate. That means that some leafy vegetables will be fine. The following 10 snack options will keep you feeling full while minimizing any effect on your blood sugar and insulin levels . . .

1) 30 grams of cheese slices
2) Celery with cream cheese
3) Cucumber boats with tuna salad
4) 5 green or back olives, stuffed with cheese
5) Half an avocado
6) Beef jerky
7) A deviled egg
8) A lettuce leaf wrapped around grated cheddar cheese
9) Sliced ham rolled around cooked French beans
10) 30 grams of nuts and seeds

Chapter 4: Beginner's Guide to Low Carb Shopping

The supermarket can be a war zone when it comes to the battle to manage your weight. In it you'll find every item you've craved, as well as all the foods you need to turn your body into a fat burning machine. Avoiding one and stock piling the other comes down to two things: preparation and discipline.

Preparation

- ✓ **Never shop on an empty stomach**. If you do, you'll make extremely unwise choices merely to satisfy your immediate urge. Have a full meal within an hour of heading to the super market to make sure that your belly doesn't rule your wallet.
- ✓ **Shop the perimeter of the store**. All supermarkets are laid out in virtually the same way. The perimeter of the store contains all the freshest foods, while the interior of the store contains all the stuff that can get you into trouble with your diet. Stay at the perimeter of the store and you can't go wrong.
- ✓ **Have a list.** Forethought is required to be able to stick to a low carb way of life. So, take the time to plan out your list before you leave home. Then stick to the list.
- ✓ **Read the Nutritional Labels.** You should view the nutritional label as the food's CV. Imagine that the food is applying to be worthy of entering your body. Be a discerning employer. If it doesn't meet your expectations, put it back. Of course, this means that you have to know what your

expectations are, so know your figures, especially the amount of carb grams per serving that you will not go beyond.

Discipline

The supermarket will test your will power to the limit. By shopping smart and sticking to the perimeter of the store, you'll by-pass many of the sugar-laden temptations, but it's when you get to the counter that they really ramp up the pressure. While you're waiting in the aisle at the counter, those mouth-watering confectionaries and chocolate bars seem to have a way of hypnotizing us. Before we know it, we've reached out and thrown one – or three – of them onto our shopping haul.

What's the solution?

It's good, old-fashioned will power. You must simply repeat the following line to yourself when you see a carb laden treat . . .

That doesn't apply to me

If you want to remain the way you are, look like the majority of people and struggle with your weight until the day you die, then give in to your food urges. If, however, you are serious about making some real traction and forging the lean and mean body that you deserve to be walking around in, get serious with yourself and don't give those unhealthy snack foods a look-in. They are not worthy of your body.

Sample Low Carb Shopping List

Proteins

1. All Fish, including herring, salmon, sardines, tuna, cod, halibut
2. All Fowl including chicken, duck, pheasant, turkey
3. All Shellfish including clams, crabmeat, mussels, oysters
4. All Meat including beef, lamb, ham, pork, venison

Dairy Products

5. Eggs
6. Butter
7. Cream
8. Sour cream
9. Cream cheese
10. Hard cheese
11. Soft cheese
12. Greek Yogurt, plain

Vegetables

13. Bell peppers
14. Broccoli
15. Cucumbers
16. Cabbage

17. Cauliflower
18. Lettuce
19. Spinach
20. Kale
21. Onions
22. Sprouts

Nuts and Seeds

23. Walnuts
24. Macadamias
25. Almonds
26. Hazelnuts
27. Pumpkin Seeds
28. Sunflower Seeds

Fruit

29. Avocado
30. Blueberries
31. Raspberries
32. Bananas

Pantry

33. Canned Tuna
34. Canned Sardines
35. Canned Tomatoes

36. Pasta, Alfredo or Pizza Sauce (no added sugar)
37. Chicken Stock
38. Vegetable Stock
39. Nut Butter

Condiments

40. Mustard
41. Cider Vinegar
42. Wine Vinegar
43. Bottled Hot Sauce
44. Soy Sauce (unless gluten sensitive)
45. Mayonnaise
46. Salad Dressing (sugar free)
47. Horseradish
48. Lemon Juice

Baking Needs

49. Whey Protein Powder
50. Splenda
51. Sugar Alcohol Sweeteners
52. Unsweetened Cocoa Powder
53. Gelatin
54. Extra-Virgin Olive Oil
55. Peanut Oil
56. Coconut Oil

57.   Sesame Oil
58.   Almond Flour

Chapter 5: Irresistible Low Carb Recipes

Low-Carb Breakfast Recipes

Protein Oatmeal Pudding

What you need:
- ✓ ½ cup of Oats
- ✓ 1 scoop of Whey Isolate Protein Powder
- ✓ ½ cup of Unsweetened Almond Milk (optional)

What you do:
1) Combine oats with the almond milk.
2) Microwave on high setting for 1-2 minutes, until the oatmeal is of a little runny consistency.
3) Add the protein powder.

Makes 1 serving.

Nutrient breakdown per serving:

Calories: 335
Carbs: 35g
Protein: 35g
Fat: 5g
Fiber: 8g

Protein Waffles

What you need:
1) 2 scoops of Whey Protein Isolate (any flavor)
2) 4 egg whites
3) ½ cup Oats, blended into flour
4) 2 packets of Stevia
5) 1 tsp. Cinnamon
6) 1 tsp. Coconut Oil

What you do:
- ✓ Beat the egg whites
- ✓ Add cinnamon, oat flour, stevia and cinnamon and mix well
- ✓ Cook on a preheated waffle maker sprayed with Pam for 3 minutes
- ✓ Meanwhile, mix all the topping ingredients
- ✓ Once the waffles are ready, pour the topping over them and enjoy!

Topping Options:
1) 2 tbsp. Almond Milk
2) 2 packets Of Stevia
3) 1 tsp. Cinnamon

Makes 2 servings.

Nutrient breakdown per serving:

Calories: 259
Carbs: 11g
Protein: 53g

Fat: 4g
Fiber: 4g

Baked Seafood Omelet

What you need:
- ✓ 100g Cooked Shrimp
- ✓ 4 egg whites
- ✓ 2 tbsp. Melted Fat Free Cottage Cheese
- ✓ ½ tsp. Tarragon
- ✓ Salt and Pepper to taste
- ✓ 1 tsp. Coconut Oil

What you do:
1) Preheat oven to 375.
2) In a bowl, whisk eggs, tarragon and cottage cheese together.
3) Pour the contents of the bowl onto a skillet oiled with coconut oil. 4. Once the omelet creates a base add the shrimp on top.
4) Place the skillet on the top shelf of the oven and bake for 5 minutes.
5) Take the omelet out of the oven, fold in half and enjoy!

Makes 1 serving.

Nutrient breakdown per serving:

Calories: 225
Carbs: 2g
Protein: 39g
Fat: 6g
Fiber: 0g

Blueberry Oatmeal Pancakes

What you need:
- ✓ ½ cup Frozen Blueberries
- ✓ 1 cup Oats
- ✓ 1 tsp. Baking Powder
- ✓ 1 cup Almond Milk (Unsweetened)
- ✓ 12 egg whites
- ✓ 1 cup Unsweetened Applesauce
- ✓ Stevia (to taste)
- ✓ 2 tsp. of Cinnamon

What you do:
1) Blend stevia, egg whites, baking powder, almond milk, salt and oats.
2) Add ¼ of the blueberries to the mixture.
3) Cook the pancakes on a lightly oiled pan over medium heat.
4) Top with a blend of applesauce, cinnamon and stevia.

Makes 1 serving.

Nutrient breakdown per serving:

Calories: 344
Carbs: 38g
Protein: 36g
Fat: 5g
Fiber: 9g

Chia Seed Cereal

What you need:
1) 1 cup of Organic Rolled Oats

2) 1 tsp. of Cinnamon
3) 1 tbsp. of Chia Seeds
4) Few drops of Stevia
5) 1 cup of Almond Milk
6) 1 scoop of Whey Protein Isolate

What you do:
- ✓ Boil/microwave the oatmeal with almond milk
- ✓ Add all the remaining ingredients

Makes 1 serving.

Nutrient breakdown per serving:

Calories: 288
Carbs: 35g
Protein: 26g
Fat: 6g
Fiber: 7.5g

Zucchini Pancakes

What you need:

1) 1 tbsp. Coconut Flour
2) 3 whole eggs
3) Sea Salt & Pepper (plus any other fresh spices and herbs to your taste)
4) 2 cups Shredded Zucchini
5) 1 tsp. Coconut Oil

What you do:
- ✓ Sift the coconut flour into the eggs and beat them together

- ✓ Mix in the shredded zucchini, sea salt & pepper
- ✓ Use a large cast iron or stainless steel skillet over medium-low heat with coconut oil coating the pan
- ✓ Spoon the mixture into the pan in size of pancake you desire
- ✓ Cook for a few minutes and flip over when golden brown

Topping ideas:
1) Unsweetened apple sauce
2) Cinnamon Nutmeg
3) Hot sauce or salsa
4) Tomato sauce
5) Caramelized onions
6) Nut butter

Chopped chives, parsley, or cilantro

Makes 1 serving.

Nutrient breakdown per serving:

Calories: 357
Carbs: 14g
Protein: 23g
Fat: 23g
Fiber: 7g

Low-Carb Lunch Recipes

Quinoa Burgers

What you need:
- ✓ 1 Large Onion
- ✓ 1 Clove Garlic
- ✓ 4 cups Broccoli
- ✓ 1 medium Zucchini

- ✓ 1 Cup Green Beans
- ✓ 1 ½ Cup of Quinoa
- ✓ 3 Cups Water
- ✓ 1 Cup Sliced Mushrooms
- ✓ 1 tsp. Coconut Oil
- ✓ 1 Lemon
- ✓ 1 Cup Quinoa Flakes
- ✓ 2 Whole Eggs – Beaten

Spice Options
Cumin, pepper, turmeric, saffron, chiliflakes

Fresh Herb Options
Basil, coriander, parsley 1 cup almond flour

What you do:

1) Place water and quinoa in a saucepan until the water boils, reduce heat, cover and simmer for 5 minutes, drain quinoa if necessary.
2) In a non-stick pan, add coconut oil, onion, garlic, selected spices and stir. Add all remaining vegetables. Once the vegetables have softened, add the quinoa, stir together. Add finely chopped selected fresh herbs and lemon juice.
3) Have 2 separate bowls ready – 1 with the beaten eggs, 1 with the almond flour and Quinoa flakes. Press the ready made quinoa into round patties and cover in egg mixture. Then roll the patties into the almond flour/Quinoa mix, as if you were making burgers.
4) You will need to have a hot, non-stick frying pan or a grill ready to cook the patties. Use 1 tsp. of coconut oil if needed.

Makes 4 servings.

Nutrient breakdown per serving:

Calories: 631
Carbs: 58g
Protein: 26g
Fat: 25g
Fiber: 15g

Serve along with Fresh **Quinoa Salad**

Low Carb Tortillas

What you need:
- ✓ 4.5 tbsp. Cottage Cheese
- ✓ 3 medium eggs
- ✓ 1 tsp. Cream of Tartar
- ✓ Pinch of Salt
- ✓ 1 tsp. Coconut Oil

What you do:
1) Blend all ingredients together until the cottage cheese is pureed and you have a smooth liquid.
2) Lightly oil a frying pan with coconut oil and heat over medium high heat.
3) Pour just enough batter in the hot skillet to coat the bottom of the pan. Once the crepe moves when you shake the pan (about 20 seconds), flip over and cook for an additional 10 seconds or until the crepe moves when you shake the pan.
4) Repeat.

Makes 3 serving.

Nutrient breakdown per serving:

Calories: 113
Carbs: 5g

Protein: 8g
Fat: 8g
Fiber: 0g

Filling ideas:

Tuna, shredded chicken, ground beef, guacamole, sour cream, cheese, salsa, egg, bacon

Serve along with **Broccoli Slaw**

Gluten Free, Low Carb, High Protein Pizza

What you need:
- ✓ 3 medium zucchini, grated
- ✓ 1 egg, & 4 egg whites
- ✓ 1 cup White Beans or Black Eyed Peas (mashed/blended to make a smooth consistency) - if you want to make this even lower in carbs use 1 cup cooked and mashed cauliflower
- ✓ Salt & pepper to your preference
- ✓ ½ cup Tomato Sauce (look for low carb/low sugar)
- ✓ 1 tsp. dry oregano
- ✓ 1 tsp. garlic powder
- ✓ ½ onion
- ✓ 2 cup spinach
- ✓ 1 cup mushrooms
- ✓ ½ red pepper
- ✓ 6 oz. chicken cooked breast
- ✓ 45g goat cheese (optional)

What you do:
1) Preheat oven to 375F.
2) Spray a pizza pan with cooking spray.

3) Mix well grated zucchini, beans (or cauliflower) with egg and egg whites (or blend together), salt and pepper

4) Place zucchini/bean mixture on the pizza pan spreading out to the edges of the pan.

5) Bake at 375F for 30 minutes.

6) Make pizza sauce by combining tomato sauce with oregano and garlic powder (add anything else you like). Spread pizza sauce on partially-cooked "crust" to within about ½ inch of the edge.

7) Dice veggies and chicken and mix with goat cheese. Add toppings to the pizza.

8) Bake for another 30 minutes or until cheese is melted and veggies are tender and cooked to your liking.

9) You can really experiment with this recipe by adding a variation of toppings and spices. Get inspirations from traditional pizza toppings and try - BBQ pizza, meat lovers etc.

10) If you use pie trays, you can simply cover with foil and store in the fridge which makes it very convenient to grab one and go.

Makes 4 servings.

Nutrient breakdown per serving:

Calories: 240
Carbs: 21g
Protein: 20g
Fat: 5g
Fiber: 17g

Serve along with **Kale and Carrot Salad**

Turkey Meatballs

What you need:
- ✓ 1 lemon - 1 tbsp. of grated lemon peel
- ✓ 2 green onions
- ✓ 2 garlic cloves
- ✓ 1 egg
- ✓ 2 tbsp. of chili garlic sauce or hot sauce
- ✓ 2 tsp. of fish sauce
- ✓ 1 lb. of ground turkey
- ✓ 3 tsp. of cornstarch
- ✓ 2 tsp. of cilantro

What you do:
1) Mix lemon grate, onion, garlic
2) Whisk egg, chili-sauce and fish sauce and add to lemon/onion/garlic mix
3) Add turkey mix in
4) Add cornstarch and cilantro
5) Make meatballs and cook for 20-30min - 400 degree

Makes 4 servings.

Nutrient breakdown per serving:

Calories: 304
Carbs: 3g
Protein: 45g
Fat: 13g
Fiber: 1g

Serve along with Mediterranean Salad (Page 48)

Baked Chicken Balls

What you need:
- ✓ 5-6 medium tomatoes
- ✓ 1 large onion
- ✓ 4lb of ground chicken
- ✓ ¼ cup fresh cilantro black pepper to taste
- ✓ salt to taste

What you do:
1) Preheat the oven for 400 Celsius.
2) Dice the tomatoes (you can buy canned ones, but I'd stay away from them, due to the preservatives).
3) Mince the onion.
4) Throw the onions and the tomatoes in a baking dish.
5) Chop up the cilantro.
6) Put the ground chicken into a bowl.
7) Throw in and mix the cilantro, black pepper and salt.
8) Make chicken balls about the size of your fist.
9) Put them in the baking dish and cook it for an hour Healthy, tasty and easy to make.

Makes approximately 14 chicken balls.

Nutrient breakdown per serving:

Calories: 321
Carbs: 3g
Protein: 49g
Fat: 13g
Fiber: 1g

Serve along with **Fresh Chicken Salad**

Chicken Spaghetti Squash

What you need:
- ✓ 1 tsp Coconut Oil
- ✓ 1 cup chopped onion
- ✓ 5 cloves minced garlic
- ✓ 1 cup sliced mushrooms
- ✓ 1 cup finely chopped fresh tomatoes
- ✓ 1 tbsp. dried basil
- ✓ ½ cup fresh parsley
- ✓ 1 tbsp. dried oregano
- ✓ 1lb extra lean ground chicken
- ✓ Salt and pepper to taste

What you do:
1) Put the ground chicken in a bowl and mix in 1 tsp. of salt, 1 tbsp. of black pepper and 1 tbsp. of garlic powder.
2) Put a skillet on medium and spray some Pam.
3) Sautee mushrooms, garlic and onion in the pan.
4) When the onions are transparent add the tomatoes, parsley, oregano and basil.
5) Set the heat on low and add 1/4 cup of water. Let the sauce simmer, while stirring occasionally.
6) In another pan, brown the chicken on medium heat. Drain any fat.
7) When the meat is done, add it to the sauce and stir everything together.
8) Serve on top of spaghetti squash.

Makes 5 servings.

Nutrient breakdown per serving:

Calories: 278

Carbs: 8g
Protein: 35g
Fat: 12g
Fiber: 1g

Serve along with **Fresh Quinoa Salad**

Lemon Curry Halibut

What you need:
- ✓ 500g of 5 fresh halibut filets (100g each)
- ✓ ¾ of lemon juice
- ✓ 1 tbsp. of chili powder
- ✓ 1 tbsp. oregano
- ✓ 1 tbsp. garlic powder
- ✓ 1 tbsp. yellow curry powder
- ✓ salt and pepper (to taste)

What you do:
1) Mix all the spices together.
2) Spray Pam on a medium heated pan.
3) Put the fillets on the pan and sprinkle them with half of the spice mix.
4) Cook for about 2 minutes.
5) Flip the fillets and sprinkle the remainder of the spice mix on top. 6. Cook until the fillets are easily flaked.

Makes 5 fillets.

Nutrient breakdown per Fillet:

Calories: 142
Carbs: 0g
Protein: 27g

Fat: 3g
Fiber: 0g

Side Dish

Baked Sweet French Fries

What you need:
- ✓ 2-3 large sweet potatoes
- ✓ 1 tsp. Coconut Oil
- ✓ 1 tsp. ground garlic
- ✓ 1 tsp. ground chili salt (to taste)

What you do:
1) Cut the potatoes into a French fry shape.
2) 2. Lightly spray them with Pam and mix.
3) 3. Add the spices and mix again.
4) 4. Place the fries on a baking dish in one layer.
5) 5. Bake for 1 hour on 375.

Makes 4 servings.

Nutrient breakdown per serving:

Calories: 72
Carbs: 20g
Protein: 2g
Fat: 2g
Fiber: 4g

Low-Carb Salad Recipes

Cucumber Radish Dill Salad

What you need:
- ✓ 1 medium cucumber
- ✓ ¼ tsp. salt
- ✓ 2 large spring onions with green stems, finely sliced
- ✓ 4 medium red radishes, thinly sliced
- ✓ ½ cup fat free Greek yogurt
- ✓ 2 tbsp. white wine vinegar
- ✓ 1 tbsp. finely chopped fresh dill or 1 tsp. dried dill
- ✓ 1 packet stevia
- ✓ 1 tsp. Dijon mustard
- ✓ ¼ tsp. freshly ground black pepper

What you do:
1) Slice cucumber in half and scoop out the seeds with a spoon.
2) 2. Place in a bowl and sprinkle with salt and let stand 30 minutes (salting cucumbers removes some of the liquid so that the flavour of a dressing is not heavily diluted).
3) 3. Drain and pat dry.
4) 4. Chop cucumber, spring onions and radishes and combine in a large bowl.
5) 5. Make dressing by combing and whisking together, vinegar, dill, stevia, mustard and pepper until combined.
6) 6. Spoon dressing over cucumber mixture and toss to coat.
7) 7. Cover and refrigerate one hour.

Makes 1 serving.

Nutrient breakdown per serving:
Calories: 118

Carbs: 21g
Protein: 21g
Fat: 0g
Fiber: 3g

Fresh Quinoa Salad

What you need:
- ✓ 1 cup quinoa
- ✓ 2 cup of water
- ✓ 1 clove of garlic, minced
- ✓ 1 medium bay leaf
- ✓ Salt and pepper (to taste)
- ✓ 1 tbsp. extra virgin olive oil
- ✓ 2 tbsp. freshly squeezed lemon juice
- ✓ 1 cup cucumber, diced ½ cup green onion

What you do:
1) Rinse quinoa in cold water for 4-5 minutes
2) Put water, garlic, bay leaf, salt and pepper in a sauce pan and bring to a boil.
3) Stir in quinoa and reduce heat to medium. Cook for about 15 minutes. Remove quinoa from heat and cool it for 15 minutes.
4) Add olive oil, lemon juice, cucumber and onion and stir well.

Makes 2 servings.

Nutrient breakdown per serving:

Calories: 282
Carbs: 43g
Protein: 10g
Fat: 5g

Fiber: 8g

Fresh Chicken Salad

What you need:
- ✓ 450g of refrigerated grilled turkey, cubed
- ✓ 3 c baby spinach
- ✓ 2 c lettuce
- ✓ 2 c fresh arugula
- ✓ 1 medium tomato, chopped
- ✓ 1 c green onion, chopped
- ✓ 4 tbsp. balsamic vinegar

What you do:
1) Toss all the ingredients into a large bowl and mix them all together.
2) Add salt and pepper to taste (optional).

Makes 3 servings.

Nutrient breakdown per serving:

Calories: 218
Carbs: 6g
Protein: 33g
Fat: 5g
Fiber: 2g

Mediterranean Salad

What you need:

- ✓ 2 cucumbers, peeled, ends cut flat, and spiralized into spaghetti noodles
- ✓ 1 cup cherry tomatoes, halved
- ✓ 1 cup kalamata olives, pitted and halved
- ✓ ½ red onion, thinly sliced
- ✓ ½ cup crumbled feta
- ✓ ½ cup olive oil
- ✓ Zest of ½ lemon, plus juice of 1 lemon
- ✓ 3 tablespoons red wine vinegar
- ✓ 2 garlic cloves, finely minced
- ✓ 1 tablespoon chopped fresh basil
- ✓ 1 table spoon chopped fresh oregano

What you do:
1) Pat the zucchini noodles dry with paper towels and out them in a large bowl.
2) Add the cherry tomatoes, olives, red onion and feta.
3) In a small bowl, whisk together the olive oil, lemon zest and juice, red wine vinegar, garlic, basil, oregano, salt, and pepper.
4) Toss the salad with the vinaigrette, or server the vinaigrette on the side for drizzling.

Makes 4 servings

Nutrients breakdown:
Calories: 351
Carbs: 13g
Protein: 5g
Fat: 33g
Fiber; 7g

Broccoli Slaw

(With creamy lemon-herb dressing and slivered almonds)

What you need:
- ✓ 2 Cup of broccoli stems, spiralized into spaghetti noodles, plus 2 cups broccoli florets
- ✓ 1 large carrot, peeled, ends cut flat, and spiralized into spaghetti noodles
- ✓ ½ cup of silvered almonds
- ✓ 1 cup Garlic Aioli
- ✓ Zest of ½ lemon, plus juice of 1 lemon
- ✓ 1 teaspoon chopped fresh rosemary
- ✓ 1 tablespoon chopped fresh thyme
- ✓ 1 tablespoon chopped fresh chives
- ✓ ½ teaspoon sea salt
- ✓ ¼ teaspoon freshly ground black pepper

What you do:
1) Cut the broccoli and carrot noodles into 2-inch pieces.
2) Put them in a large bowl and add the broccoli florets and almonds.
3) In a small bowl, whisk together the aioli, lemon zest and juice, rosemary, thyme, chives, salt, and pepper
4) Toss the salad with the dressing.

Makes 4 servings

Nutrient breakdown per serving:

Calories: 343
Carbs: 26g
Protein: 6g
Fat: 26g
Fiber: 5g

Beet and Arugula Salad
(with goat cheese and walnuts)

What you need:
- ✓ 1 pound beets, peeled, ends cut flat, and spiralized, into spaghetti noodles
- ✓ 2 cups baby arugula
- ✓ 1 shallot, thinly sliced
- ✓ ½ cup goat cheese
- ✓ ¼ cup walnut pieces
- ✓ ½ cup olive oil
- ✓ 3 tablespoons balsamic vinegar
- ✓ 1 tablespoon Dijon mustard
- ✓ 2 tablespoons chapped fresh tarragon
- ✓ ½ teaspoon sea salt
- ✓ ¼ teaspoon freshly ground black pepper

What you do:
1) In a large bowl, combine the beet noodles, carrot noodles, baby arugula, shallot, goat cheese, and walnuts.
2) In a small bowl, whisk together the olive oil, vinegar, mustard, tarragon, salt, and pepper.
3) Toss the dressing with the salad, or serve it on the side for drizzling.

Make 4 servings

Nutrient breakdown per serving:
Calories:380
Carbs: 16g
Protein: 7g
Fat: 34g
Fiber: 4g

Carrot and Kale Salad

What you need:
- ✓ 2 large carrots, peeled, ends cut flat, and spiralized into spaghetti noodles
- ✓ 4 cups torn deribbed kale
- ✓ ¼ cup pine nuts
- ✓ For the Vinaigrette
- ✓ 3 tablespoons balsamic vinegar
- ✓ 1 teaspoon Dijon mustard
- ✓ ¼ cup olive oil
- ✓ ½ teaspoon sea salt
- ✓ ¼ teaspoon freshly ground black pepper
- ✓ Zest and juice of 1 orange
- ✓ ¼ teaspoon Sriracha
- ✓ 1 garlic clove, minced

What you do:

1) Cut the carrot noodles cross-wise into 2-inch pieces.
2) Put them in a large bowl and add the kale and pine nuts.
3) In a small bowl, whisk together the balsamic vinegar, Dijon mustard, olive oil, salt, pepper, orange zest and juice, sriracha, and garlic.
4) Toss the salad with the vinaigrette, or serve it on for drizzling.

Make 4 servings

Nutrient breakdown per serving:
Calories:254
Carbs: 14g
Protein: 4g
Fat: 3g

Fiber: 2g

Creamy Chicken Salad

What you need:
- ✓ 2 large carrots, peels, ends cut flat, and spiralized into ribboned noodles
- ✓ 1 cup broccoli florets
- ✓ 1 red bell pepper, seeded and cut into matchsticks
- ✓ ½ fennel bulb, shaved with vegetable peeler or mandolin
- ✓ 2 scallions, thinly sliced
- ✓ 4 cups chopped, cooked chicken
- ✓ ½ cup garlic aioli
- ✓ Grated zest of ½ lemon, plus 1 tablespoon freshly squeezed lemon juice
- ✓ 2 tablespoons chopped fresh tarragon
- ✓ ½ teaspoon sea salt
- ✓ ¼ teaspoon freshly ground black pepper

What you do:
1) Cut the carrot ribbons cross-wise into 2-inch pieces.
2) Put them in a large bowl and add the broccoli, bell pepper, fennel, scallions and chicken.
3) In a small bowl, whisk together the aioli, lemon zest and juice, tarragon, salt and pepper.
4) Toss the salad with the dressing and serve.

Make 4 servings

Nutrient breakdown per serving:
Calories:313
Carbs: 10g
Protein: 43g

Fat: 3g
Fiber: 3g

Low-Carb Dinners Meal Recipes

Chicken Shawarma Lettuce Wraps

- ✓ What you need:
- ✓ 1 cup shredded English cucumber
- ✓ ¼ cup non-fat plain Greek yogurt
- ✓ 1 tbsp. tahini
- ✓ 2 tbsp.s lemon juice
- ✓ ½ tsp. salt, divided
- ✓ 1 tbsp. garlic powder
- ✓ 1 tsp. curry powder
- ✓ ½ tsp. freshly ground pepper
- ✓ 1 pound boneless, skinless chicken breast, trimmed
- ✓ 1 tbsp. coconut oil
- ✓ Large romaine lettuce leaves

What you do:
1) Preheat grill to medium.
2) Stir cucumber, yogurt, tahini, lemon juice and 1/4 tsp. salt together in a medium bowl. Set aside.
3) Combine garlic powder, curry powder, pepper and the remaining 1/4 tsp. salt in another medium bowl. Slice chicken breast crosswise into 1/4-inch strips; toss with the spice mixture to coat. Add 1 tbsp. oil and toss to combine.
4) Grill the chicken, turning once, until cooked through, about 2 minutes per side.

5) To serve, spread 1/4 cup of the cucumber-yogurt sauce on a large lettuce leaf and top with one-fourth of the chicken. Fold like a taco and enjoy!

Makes 2 servings.

Nutrient breakdown per serving:

Calories: 257
Carbs: 4g
Protein: 39g
Fat: 9g
Fiber: 0g

Carb Free "Sushi"

What you need:
- ✓ 2-3 Roasted Seaweed Nori Sheets
- ✓ 1 can of low-sodium white tuna (in water)
- ✓ 2 tbsp. low-sodium fermented soy sauce
- ✓ ½ tsp. sesame oil(optional)
- ✓ 2 tbsp. chopped green onions
- ✓ 1 tsp. chili powder 2 + 2 tbsp.
- ✓ Fat Free Mayo
- ✓ 2 Tbsp. Rice vinegar
- ✓ ¼ cucumber (cut lengthwise into match sticks)

What you do:
1) Mix tuna, soy sauce, sesame oil, green onion, chili powder
2) 2 tbsp. mayo, and rice vinegar together in a bowl.
3) Lay nori sheets flat one by one on a cutting board. Spread 1 tbsp. mayo to cover the entire sheet in a thin layer. This will soften the nori sheet so they don't break and allow you to get them to stick when you roll them.

4) Add tuna mixture in the center lengthwise.
5) Add cucumber matchsticks.
6) Add wasabi if desired.
7) Roll nori sheets into a tube/wrap style. Best to eat like a wrap or hand roll (if you choose to cut into maki style, use a very sharp knife and make sure the wrap is very tight.
8) You can also get some pickled ginger and have it on the side.

Makes 1 serving.

Nutrient breakdown per serving

Calories: 221
Carbs: 4g
Protein: 5g
Fat: 9g
Fiber: 0g

Chicken Tacos Salad

What you need:
- ✓ 300g of extra lean ground chicken or turkey
- ✓ ½ large yellow onion chopped
- ✓ ½ red pepper chopped
- ✓ 1 tsp. oregano
- ✓ 2 tsp. chili pepper
- ✓ ½ tsp. black pepper
- ✓ 1 packet stevia
- ✓ 1 small can of diced tomatoes drained
- ✓ Salt to taste
- ✓ 6 leaves of romaine lettuce

What you do:

1) Spray a medium sized pot with PAM and heat on mid high heat.
2) Add onions and peppers and cook until onions are transparent.
3) Add all other ingredients except for canned tomatoes and lettuce
4) Mix everything together in the pot and cook until the ground chicken/turkey is done.
5) Remove from heat and drain any excess liquid.
6) Bring it back on the stovetop, reduce heat to medium low and add the canned tomatoes.
7) Cook an additional 5 minutes. Remove from stove and serve.
8) You can use romaine leaves as "taco" shells and add chicken mixture inside each leaf or simply chop up the lettuce and add mixture on top and serve as a salad.

Makes 2 servings.

Nutrient breakdown per serving:

Calories: 220
Carbs: 8g
Protein: 29g
Fat: 15g
Fiber: 3g

Chicken Meatloaf

What you need:
- ✓ 2.5lb of extra lean ground chicken
- ✓ 1 medium onion
- ✓ 1 green pepper
- ✓ ½ c zucchini
- ✓ ½ c broccoli

- ✓ 2 stems of celery
- ✓ 1 c mushrooms
- ✓ 1 tbsp. thyme
- ✓ ¼ c fresh basil
- ✓ ¼ c fresh parsley
- ✓ salt and pepper (to taste)
- ✓ 4 egg whites
- ✓ 2 c organic rolled oats
- ✓ 1 clove minced garlic

What you do:
1) In a skillet sprayed with Pam, sauté onions, pepper, zucchini, broccoli, celery and mushrooms until tender.
2) Add garlic 1-2 minutes before the vegetables are done, remove from heat and cool them off for about 5 minutes.
3) In a large bowl, mix the rest of the ingredients with the sautéed vegetables.
4) Put the mixture into loaf pans or any baking dish sprayed with Pam.
5) Put in an oven on 425 degrees Celsius for 40 minutes.
6) Remove from the oven and let the meatloaf sit for 45 minutes.
7) Slice into 8 pieces and enjoy.

Makes 8 servings.

Nutrient breakdown per serving:

Calories: 288
Carbs: 19g
Protein: 32g
Fat: 16g
Fiber: 3g

Grilled Chicken Breast with Veggie Salsa

What you need:
- ✓ 2 4oz Chicken Breasts
- ✓ 2 cups Cherry tomatoes
- ✓ 2 cups Zucchini
- ✓ 1 cup Broccoli
- ✓ 2 tbsp. Coriander
- ✓ 2 c. Celery
- ✓ 1 clove Garlic, minced
- ✓ 1 cup Onion
- ✓ 2 cups Mushrooms
- ✓ 1 tsp. Ginger
- ✓ 1 tsp. Chili
- ✓ Lime Juice, to taste

What you do:
1) Grill Chicken breast until cooked through
2) Using a non-stick pan add garlic, onion, chili, lime juice, ginger, mushrooms, zucchini, and cherry tomatoes.
3) Once they have cooked add the broccoli and celery and cook for additional 3-5 minutes, leaving the greens a little bit crunchy.
4) Add the coriander and more lime juice as required.

Makes 2 servings.

Nutrient breakdown per serving:

Calories: 250
Carbs: 37g
Protein: 33g
Fat: 2g
Fiber: 8g

Mexican Rissoles on a Layer of Salsa

What you need:
For Salsa:
- ✓ Finely chopped: 1 medium tomato
- ✓ Finely chopped: ¼ of large cucumber
- ✓ Finely chopped: ¼ red onion
- ✓ half avocado
- ✓ juice from ½ a lime
- ✓ chili powder to taste
- ✓ Iceberg lettuce

For Rissoles:
- ✓ 500g of ground beef
- ✓ 1 chopped medium onion
- ✓ 2 cloves of garlic minced
- ✓ ¼ cup of almond meal
- ✓ chili to taste

What you do:
1) Dice all salsa ingredients, mix in a bowl and refrigerate.
2) Sautee onion and let it cool.
3) Mix in a bowl beef, almond meal and chili.
4) Once your onion has cooled down add it to the mix and mix everything together.
5) Roll the mixture into 10 balls and cook on a low heat in the pan sprayed with Pam.
6) Put a layer of Salsa on a lettuce leaf.
7) Add 3 rissoles and enjoy!

Makes 5 serving.

Nutrient breakdown per serving:

Calories: 423
Carbs: 8g
Protein: 36g
Fat: 25g
Fiber: 3g

Turkey Breast Fast Wraps

What you need:
- ✓ 50g thinly sliced smoked turkey breast.
- ✓ 30g Allegro cheese, shredded
- ✓ Iceberg Lettuce Leaves
- ✓ Broccoli sprouts
- ✓ ½ thinly sliced avocado
- ✓ Cayenne pepper

What you do:
1) Put all the ingredients into the lettuce wraps and add Cayenne pepper at the very end.
2) Enjoy!

Makes 1 serving.

Nutrient breakdown per serving:

Calories: 370
Carbs: 18g
Protein: 26g
Fat: 24g
Fiber: 3g

Grilled Tomato Shrimp

What you need:
- ✓ 2 cloves garlic, minced
- ✓ 4 tbsp. olive oil
- ✓ 1 medium tomato, cubed
- ✓ 1 tbsp. red wine
- ✓ vinegar 2 tbsp.
- ✓ fresh basil, chopped
- ✓ Salt and pepper (to taste)
- ✓ 1lb of fresh peeled shrimp

What you do:
1) Combine garlic, olive oil, tomato, vinegar, basil, salt and pepper in a blender.
2) Pour the mixture into a bowl and add the shrimp.
3) Put the bowl in the refrigerator for an hour.
4) Preheat the grill on medium heat.
5) Place the shrimp on skewers.
6) Spray Pam on the grill and grill the shrimp for 2 minutes on each side.

Makes 2 servings.

Nutrient breakdown per serving:

Calories: 327
Carbs: 2g
Protein: 32g
Fat: 20g
Fiber: 0g

Grilled Balsamic Basa

What you need:
- ✓ 4 100g basa fillets
- ✓ 1 tbsp. fresh rosemary, chopped
- ✓ Salt and pepper (to taste)
- ✓ ½ c balsamic vinegar
- ✓ 1 tbsp. extra virgin olive oil
- ✓ 4 tbsp. lemon juice, freshly squeezed
- ✓ 4 c baby spinach

What you do:
1) In a bowl, combine the vinegar, lemon juice and olive oil.
2) Pour the marinade over the salmon and refrigerate for 1.5 hours. 3. Remove from the fridge and sprinkle spices and rosemary over the fish.
3) Grill for about 5 minutes on each side, until the fillets start to flake.
4) Serve over baby spinach.

Makes 4 servings.

Nutrient breakdown per serving:

Calories: 282
Carbs: 2g
Protein: 32g
Fat: 18g
Fiber: 2g

Tuna Cucumber Roll

What you need:
- ✓ ¼ English cucumber
- ✓ 1 can tuna
- ✓ ½ avocado
- ✓ 2 tbsp. of mustard (yellow or Dijon)
- ✓ salt and pepper (to taste)

What you do:
1) In a bowl, mix tuna, mustard and avocado.
2) Cut the cucumber into ½ inch thick slices.
3) Discard the centers of the cucumber slices (either cut them out with a knife, or push them out with your fingers).
4) Stuff the hollow centered cucumbers with the tuna mix.
5) Add salt and pepper and enjoy!

Makes 1 serving.

Nutrient breakdown per serving:

Calories: 394
Carbs: 13g
Protein: 33g
Fat: 24g
Fiber: 10g

Tom Yum Soup

What you need:
- ✓ 6 cups organic chicken/beef or vegetable stock
- ✓ 2 tbsp. frozen prepared lemongrass
- ✓ 3-4 lime leaves
- ✓ 3-4 cloves garlic minced
- ✓ 1 thumb-size piece of ginger

✓ 3 tbsp. fish sauce or 4 tbsp. soy sauce (use wheat-free soy sauce for gluten-free diets)
✓ 1 tbsp. fresh lime juice
✓ 1 fresh red chili, or ½ tsp. dried crushed chili vegetables of your choice (mushrooms, cauliflower, bok choy, broccoli)
✓ 30 shrimp or 3 chicken breasts (cooked)
✓ ½ can coconut milk
✓ ½ cup fresh basil and/or ½ cup fresh coriander (cilantro)

What you do:
1) Combine first 4 ingredients together and let boil.
2) Bring the heat to low-medium and add everything except the last 3 ingredients.
3) Simmer for 15 minutes or so (until the vegetables are cooked to your liking).
4) Add coconut milk and your meat.
5) Let cook another 3-5 minutes (until it lightly bubbles again).
6) For final touch top off with cilantro or basil when serving in bowls.

Makes 2 servings.

Nutrient breakdown per serving:

Calories: 261
Carbs: 8g
Protein: 32g
Fat: 12g
Fiber: 3g

Bun-Less Mushroom Cheese Burgers

What you need:
✓ 500g of extra lean ground turkey

- ✓ 3 oz. Allegro 4% cheese, chopped
- ✓ ½ cup sun-dried tomatoes, drained and chopped
- ✓ 2 cloves garlic, minced
- ✓ 2 tsp. cumin powder
- ✓ 8 large Portobello mushrooms (stem removed) for "burger buns"
- ✓ cooking spray

What you do:
1) Combine first five ingredients together in a large bowl. Lightly mix together and form into 4 patties.
2) Heat a large pan over medium high add oil or cooking spray and cook the patties about 5-6 minutes on each side (lightly cut in the middle to make sure they are fully cooked). Remove from heat.
3) Clean the pan and add oil or cooking spray again and grill the Portobello mushrooms several minutes on each side until tender. Remove from heat.
4) Place each of the burger patties on a grilled mushroom cap, add shredded cabbage and use other burger toppings you wish.
5) Place second mushroom cap on top.

Makes 4 servings.
Nutrient Breakdown Per 1 Serving:

Calories: 249
Carbs: 15g
Protein: 34g
Fat: 7g
Fiber: 3g

Grilled Tomato Shrimp

What you need:
- ✓ 2 cloves garlic, minced
- ✓ 4 tbsp. olive oil
- ✓ 1 medium tomato, cubed
- ✓ 1 tbsp. red wine vinegar
- ✓ 2 tbsp. fresh basil, chopped
- ✓ Salt and pepper (to taste)
- ✓ 1lb of fresh peeled shrimp

What you do:
1) Combine garlic, olive oil, tomato, vinegar, basil, salt and pepper in a blender.
2) Pour the mixture into a bowl and add the shrimp.
3) Put the bowl in the refrigerator for an hour.
4) Preheat the grill on medium heat.
5) Place the shrimp on skewers.
6) Spray Pam on the grill and grill the shrimp for 2 minutes on each side. Enjoy this delicious dish with the side dish of your choice.

Makes 2 servings.

Nutrient breakdown per serving:

Calories: 327
Carbs: 2g
Protein: 32g
Fat: 20g
Fiber: 0g

Breadless Crab Cakes

What you need:
- ✓ 8oz crab meat, canned

- ✓ 2 egg whites
- ✓ 2 tsp. Worcestershire sauce
- ✓ 1 tbsp. freshly squeezed lemon juice
- ✓ 1 tsp. Tarragon
- ✓ Salt and pepper (to taste)

What you do:
1) Turn oven to broil.
2) In a bowl, mix egg whites, and seasonings.
3) Divide the mixture in two and shape them into two balls.
4) Put the crab balls into a baking dish sprayed with pam and broil for 8 minutes
5) Remove from oven, cool it, and enjoy it!

Makes 2 servings.

Nutrient breakdown per serving

Calories: 118
Carbs: 5g
Protein: 26g
Fat: 0g
Fiber: 0g

Low-Carb Cookies & Desserts

Apple Cinnamon Protein Muffins

What you need:
- ✓ 2 cups Oats
- ✓ ½ cup of Oat Bran
- ✓ 12 Egg whites

- ✓ 1 scoop of Vanilla Protein Powder
- ✓ ½ tsp. of Baking Soda
- ✓ 5 packets stevia
- ✓ 2 diced Apples
- ✓ 4 Tbsp. of Unsweetened Apple Sauce
- ✓ 1 tsp. of Cinnamon
- ✓ 1 tsp. of Vanilla Extract

What you do:
1) Preheat the oven for 350 degrees.
2) In a blender, blend all the ingredients (except for the diced apple), until mixture is thick.
3) Add the diced apple and stir (with a spoon or a spatula).
4) Poor the mix in a muffin cooking pan, and bake at 350 for approximately 30 minutes.

Makes 6 large muffins.

Nutrient breakdown per serving:

Calories: 203
Carbs: 32g
Protein: 18g
Fat: 2g
Fiber: 5g

Homemade Gluten Free, Healthy Protein Bars

What you need:
- ✓ 6 tbsp. unsweetened shredded coconut
- ✓ 6 tbsp.¼ cup almond flour (buy at a health food store or make your own by blending almonds)

- ✓ ½ cup ground flax seeds
- ✓ 1/3 cup chopped walnuts
- ✓ ¼ cup natural sweetener like Stevia
- ✓ 8 scoops chocolate whey protein powder
- ✓ 4 large table spoons of natural almond butter
- ✓ ½ cup unsweetened almond milk

What you do:

1) Mix all dry ingredients together. Add almond butter and mix until everything sticks together. Finally, add a bit of almond milk slowly until you get a good sticky mix (not too gooey) just enough so you can form it into a big flat pancake shape that wont fall apart.
2) Spray some non stick oil-spray into a square or rectangular pan, and sprinkle shredded coconut at the bottom.
3) Spread the mix onto the pan, you may have to use your hands. 4. Finally, sprinkle with some more shredded coconut on top as well so that it's not too sticky later.
4) Refrigerate for a few hours, and when the mixture is nice and firm, cut into squares.

Makes 8 bars.

Nutrient breakdown per serving:

Calories: 313
Carbs: 9g
Protein: 33g
Fat: 16g
Fiber: 6g

Protein Cupcakes

What you need:
- ✓ 8 egg whites

- ✓ 1 scoop of protein powder (banana flavor is the best)
- ✓ 1tbsp of cocoa powder
- ✓ 1tsp cinnamon
- ✓ ¼ cup oat bran
- ✓ 3-4 packets of stevia

What you do:
1) Preheat the oven to 350
2) Mix the egg whites, protein powder, cinnamon, stevia and the cocoa powder together in a blender.
3) Pour the mixture in a cupcake dish, filling ¾ of each socket.
4) Bake for 30 minutes. The cupcakes should be very fluffy and puff out of their sockets.
5) Take out of the oven and cook for 10 minutes
6) Enjoy!

Makes 2 servings.

Nutrient breakdown per serving:

Calories: 161
Carbs: 11g
Protein: 31g
Fat: 2g
Fiber: 3g

Gluten, Carb and Dairy Free Bread

What you need:
- ✓ 300g almond meal
- ✓ 4 tbsp. olive oil
- ✓ 1 tsp. baking powder
- ✓ 6 egg whites
- ✓ stevia to taste

✓ 2 tsp. of cinnamon

What you do:
1) Mix all the ingredients together to make a dough.
2) Form into a loaf shape into your baking tin.
3) Bake for around 30min on 200 degrees Celsius.
4) Let the loaf cool for 20 minutes and remove from tin.
5) Enjoy!

Makes 10 servings.

Nutrient Breakdown Per serving:

Calories: 236
Carbs: 7g
Protein: 21g
Fat: 9g
Fiber: 3g

Homemade Protein Bars

What you need:
✓ 2 ½ c. (200 g) oats
✓ 2 scoop (30 g) whey protein isolate (use chocolate flavor)
✓ 6 egg whites
✓ 2 medium bananas (300 g) mashed
✓ 1 tbsp. Honey
✓ ½ cup almond milk
✓ 1 tsp. Cinnamon

What you do:
1) Preheat the oven to 355.
2) Mix together the oats, whey and cinnamon.
3) Add egg whites, mashed bananas and honey.

4) Add lactose free skim milk slowly while mixing.
5) Spoon the mixture into a lined cake tin sprayed with Pam and level with a knife.
6) Place in oven and bake for 15 minutes.
7) Remove from oven and allow to cook for 5 minutes.
8) Cut into 4 bars.

Makes 4 bars.

Nutrient breakdown for 1 bar:

Calories: 329
Carbs: 54g
Protein: 28g
Fat: 4g
Fiber: 5g

Protein Cinnamon Cake with Cocoa Syrup

What you need:
- ✓ 5 scoops of protein powder
- ✓ 8 egg whites
- ✓ 1-2 tbsp. of cinnamon
- ✓ ¼ tsp. of baking powder
- ✓ 1 tsp. vanilla extract
- ✓ Stevia to taste
- ✓ 100ml of water
- ✓ 1 tbsp. cocoa powder

What you do:
Cake:
1) Mix the dry ingredients in a blender.
2) Add the egg whites to the mix.

3) Slowly add water. You are looking for a smooth consistency, the mixture should not be runny.
4) Pour the mixture into a microwave friendly dish and cover.
5) Microwave for 4 minutes.
6) Cool the cake for 10-15 minutes.

Syrup:
1) Mix stevia, cocoa powder and 1 tsp. of cinnamon
2) Add a few drops of water. Very little, so the consistency is not runny.
3) Pour it on top of the cake
4) Serve and Enjoy!

Makes 5 servings.

Nutrient breakdown per serving:

Calories: 145
Carbs: 2g
Protein: 33g
Fat: 0g
Fiber: 0g

"Get Jacked" Frozen Yogurt

What you need:
✓ ¾ cup of Greek yogurt
✓ 1 tbsp. crushed flax seeds
✓ 1 scoop whey protein isolate (any flavor)
✓ Stevia (optional)
✓ Carb and fat free pudding powder

What you do:
1) Mix all the ingredients together.

2) Put in the freezer for 2-3 hours.
3) Take out and enjoy!

Makes 2 servings.

Nutrient breakdown per serving:

Calories: 123
Carbs: 5g
Protein: 24g
Fat: 2g
Fiber: 2g

Blueberry Cookies

What you need:
- ✓ 8 egg whites
- ✓ 1 cup blueberries
- ✓ 1 cup oat flour (simply blend the oats in a blender)
- ✓ 2 scoops of whey isolate protein powder (vanilla works best)
- ✓ ¼ tsp. baking powder

What you do:
1) Combine all the ingredients, except blueberries, in a bowl and mix well.
2) Add the blueberries and mix them with the rest of the ingredients.
3) Spoon the dough and put it on a baking dish (should make 20 cookies).
4) Bake on 375 F for 12 minutes or until crispy.

Makes 20 cookies.

Nutrient breakdown per serving:

Calories: 41
Carbs: 4g
Protein: 5g
Fat: 0g
Fiber: 1g

Cinnamon Oatmeal High Protein Frozen Pudding

What you need:
- ✓ ½ cup oatmeal
- ✓ 1 scoop of favorite Whey Protein Powder (Vanilla or Chocolate flavor)
- ✓ 3 packets of Stevia
- ✓ Cinnamon

What you do:
1) Mix all of the ingredients into a bowl.
2) Add water.
3) Place in the freezer to cool for 30 to 60 min.
4) Enjoy your high protein frozen pudding.

Makes 1 serving.

Nutrient breakdown per serving:

Calories: 305
Carbs: 33g
Protein: 34g
Fat: 4g
Fiber: 5g

Veggie and Egg Muffins

What you need:
- ✓ 1 lb. mushrooms (thinly sliced)
- ✓ 3 cups steamed broccoli (cut into small pieces)
- ✓ 150 g Allégro Cheese (4% - any flavor – grated)
- ✓ 4 green onions (chopped)
- ✓ 1 tsp. Italian Seasoning
- ✓ 1 tsp. garlic powder
- ✓ Salt & pepper to taste
- ✓ 1.5 tsp. olive oil
- ✓ 6 whole eggs
- ✓ 6 egg whites
- ✓ Muffin tray

What you do:
1) Preheat over at 350°F.
2) In the meantime spray a large pan with non-stick spray, and sauté mushrooms and onions on high heat until browned.
3) While the mushrooms are cooking, place steamed broccoli in large bowl, add olive oil, Italian seasoning and garlic powder and mash with a fork until chunky.
4) Once the mushrooms are done, add them to the broccoli, mix and set aside to cool.
5) Once room temperature add the grated cheese salt and pepper.
6) Spray muffin tray with non-stick cooking spray and add the broccoli, mushroom, cheese mixture ¾ full (should have enough for 6 muffins).
7) Now beat eggs and egg whites in a bowl until fluffy, add salt and pepper.
8) Pour egg mixture over the vegetables in the muffin tin.
9) Bake 10-15 minutes (until eggs set on top).
10) Enjoy! (these can be refrigerated or frozen for later use)

Makes 6 servings.
Nutrient breakdown per serving:

Calories: 187
Carbs: 10g
Protein: 23g
Fat: 7g
Fiber: 2g

Zucchini Chips with Cajun Dip

What you need:
For the Chips
- ✓ 2 large zucchini
- ✓ 1 tbsp. olive oil
- ✓ ¼ tsp. salt
- ✓ ½ tsp. garlic powder
- ✓ ½ tsp. chili powder

For the dip
- ✓ 1 cup low fat cottage cheese
- ✓ 1.5 tbsp. Cajun Seasoning

What you do:
1) Preheat oven at 400°F.
2) In the meantime, slice zucchini approximately 1/8 of an inch thick.
3) Place in a large bowl and toss with olive oil, salt, garlic powder, and chili powder.
4) Spray a large baking sheet (you may need two) with nonstick cooking spray like PAM, and arrange zucchini slices in a single layer.
5) Bake for 25mins turning often.

6) Reduce temperature to 300°F and bake until crisp (another 10-15mins).
7) While the zucchini is baking make the dip by mixing Cajun Seasoning with cottage cheese and place in fridge until ready to use.
8) Once the zucchini is baked, remove from oven and place on paper towels and let it cool.

Makes 3 servings of dip and zucchini chips.

Nutrient breakdown per serving:

Calories: 65
Carbs: 5g
Protein: 8g
Fat: 2g
Fiber: 1g

Protein Fudge Balls

What You Need:
- ✓ 3 scoops of chocolate whey protein powder
- ✓ 1 cup almond meal
- ✓ 50g desiccated coconut plus 10g extra for coating
- ✓ 1 tsp. peanut butter
- ✓ 50g unsweetened cocoa
- ✓ 4 packets Stevia
- ✓ Cold water

What You Do:
1) Combine all ingredients except water and additional coconut for coating.
2) Knead together into a paste, gradually adding water until it is dough-like.

3) Mold into 21 small balls and cover in additional coconut.

Makes 21 fudge balls.

Nutrient breakdown per serving (3 fudge balls):

Calories: 230
Carbs: 9g
Protein: 17g
Fat: 15g
Fiber: 6g

High Protein Cheesecake

What you need:
- ✓ ¾ cup nonfat cottage cheese
- ✓ 2/3 cup nonfat plain yogurt
- ✓ 1 tbsp. oat flour
- ✓ 5 packets stevia
- ✓ ¼ tsp. salt
- ✓ 4 egg whites
- ✓ Juice from ½ a lemon
- ✓ ½ cup blueberries
- ✓ 1oz chopped pecans (optional)

What you do:
1) Preheat oven to 350° F.
2) 2. Blend cottage cheese, yogurt, oat flour, stevia, salt and lemon juice in a blender until smooth and creamy.
3) 3. Add egg whites to the mixture and pulse a few times.
4) 4. Remove blender from the base and add the berries and stir in the mixture with a spoon (do not blend the berries).
5) 5. Spray the bottom of your pan (or use muffin tin) with some cooking spray and line with chopped pecans for crust.

6) 6. Pour the batter mixture in.
7) Bake for approximately 30 minutes checking frequently to make sure the cheesecake does not brown or dry out.
8) Chill the cake in the fridge for a few hours.

Makes 4 servings.

Nutrient breakdown per serving:

Calories: 146
Carbs: 12g
Protein: 17g
Fat: 5g
Fiber: 2g

Blueberry Ice Cream

What you need:
- ✓ 1 cup fat free cottage cheese
- ✓ 1/3 cup frozen blueberries Stevia (to taste)
- ✓ 1 tsp. natural vanilla extract
- ✓ ¼ cup of unsweetened almond milk

What you do:
1) Blend all the ingredients to form a paste.
2) Put it in a bowl and enjoy

You can also make a smoothie out of the same ingredients. Simply, add 1 extra cup of unsweetened almond milk.

Makes 1 serving.

Nutrient breakdown per serving:

Calories: 234
Carbs: 22g
Protein: 32g
Fat: 1g
Fiber: 1g

Chapter 6: Managing Cravings for Snack Foods

Food carvings come about when we have to satisfy an emotional need. When most people have strong cravings, it is for carbohydrates. Invariably it's the cookies, the crackers, or the cream cake that they reach for. What's going on is that the carbohydrates boost the level of serotonin that is in the brain. When that's increased our bodies undergo a calming effect – it de-stresses us.

A big step in overcoming food cravings, then, involves finding better ways to relieve our stress. Have you ever been in a situation where you've had to have a specific type of cake or cookie? It's probably because your body is undergoing some sort of stress. The brain has a reward center. When we eat certain types of food, we feel good. Our reward center will remember what food it is that makes us feel good and that is what we will crave when the stress comes in on us. So, when it comes to cravings think about the things that are going on in your life that are causing stress.

Here are 5 sure-fire ways that you can control your cravings:

- ✓ **Seek and Destroy** – You don't want the craving to control you; you need to control it. That means that you need to seek and destroy the temptation. So do whatever it takes to terminate that treat – crumble it up, pour water on it, tip it out, it doesn't matter. If it's in your house, you have to destroy it. You may have bought it as a treat, reasoning that you'll have it in moderation. But when that craving hits, moderation will go out the window, along with your clean eating plans!

✓ **Distract Yourself** – A craving usually lasts 10-15 minutes. In that time period, you can go take a walk, you can call a friend, you can run an errand, do push ups or shoot baskets. Whatever it is, make sure that you do something to get your mind off the craving. A craving comes like a big crashing wave. It will eventually subside.

✓ **Indulge a little bit** – You can have something that you really want, but you must have a small amount. Plan for the treat by cutting back on your carbs and total calories earlier in the day. Of course not everybody has the will power to stop after the first small slice.

✓ **Brush Your Teeth** – When you have a minty taste in your mouth, your desire for your crave food will diminish markedly. Brushing your teeth or gargling could be just what you need to stop you reaching for the donut.

✓ **Try Healthy Alternatives** – If you are craving chocolate, for example, there are certain chocolate alternatives that you can take that will satisfy the crave with the carbs. Consider using fruits and vegetables with a side of dip. Make recipes ahead of time. You should also drink a full glass of water when a craving comes on. The brain will often mistake thirst for hunger.

✓ **Chew Gum** - Carry around a packet of sugar-free gum. If you feel yourself getting a craving, chew gum. As mentioned previously in regards to brushing your teeth, the mint in gum will help cut any cravings you have.

Beat Cravings With a Food Diary

Keeping a food diary is an effective craving control method. A food diary is a list of the foods and beverages you consume throughout the day. Once you've completed your daily food diary, you'll be able to analyze it and see what foods are causing you to gain weight, what foods are missing from your diet and what situations and emotions triggered eating.

Rather than filling out your food diary as you eat your foods during the course of the day, though, leave the task until the evening. In fact, make a little ritual out of it. Get yourself comfortable on the couch with your food diary, your water bottle and an online calorie calculator. As you begin recalling and recording what you've eaten throughout the day, you will proceed with the mindset that your eating for the day is done and is now being recorded for posterity. You are now looking back on your day's eating – there is no way that you are going to add anything new to your list; it doesn't work that way!

As you write down the foods that you've eaten, also record how you were feeling at the time you ate them, along with the situation you were in. If you identify that, during times of stress, you are eating more than the usual amount or you're eating junk food, you can probably identify yourself as an emotional eater. An emotional eater is someone who eats in response to stress.

Once you have listed the foods that you've eaten, along with the way you felt and the situation you were in, you will now be able to identify your psychological triggers. Psychological triggers are situations that cause certain behaviors on your part.

So, what can you do with this information? If you know that you are going to face a stressful situation, you can either avoid the situation all together, or substitute another behavior, i.e. instead of watching TV, read a book.

In conjunction with analyzing the emotional and situational factors associated with your eating, you can benefit greatly by tracking your calorie consumption by way of your food diary. In fact, many experts belief that tracking your calories is the single most important thing you can do to improve your eating habits. There are a number of ways to easily and conveniently track your calories. The first is by using a mobile app. A great app that makes it really easy to input your foods and keep track of how many calories you're consuming is **Lose It.**

You can download **Lose It** here . . .

(https://www.loseit.com/)

Of course, you may prefer to record your calories the old school way, which is in your food diary, along with the information we've already discussed. You can use a whole host of websites to find the calorie content of the foods you eat.

Most calorie counting recommendations suggest that you only do so, for a week, or two at most. However, the very act of sitting down and thinking about what you've been eating is a great psychological aid to weight control. Sitting down and going over your good, and possibly not so good, food choices throughout the day is going to make you very unlikely to reach for any extra calories. That's why you should get into the food diary habit and set aside time every night to contemplate your daily caloric consumption.

Action Plan:

Step One

Go out and purchase yourself an attractive food diary. Keep it in a handy spot and take pride in completing it every day.

Step Two

As you go through your day, remember that you will be recording what you're about to eat in the food diary. How will you explain that chocolate chip muffin to yourself tonight?

Step Three

Have a set time each night when you sit down and complete your food diary. Put on some soothing music, put your feet up and enjoy this time to do something just for you. Have your water bottle with you and sip from it as you complete your diary.

Step Four

Analyze the results of your food diary. Identify trends in terms of situational and emotional eating. Look for ways that you make changes in order to overcome any unwise eating choices that you have identified.

Step Five

Work out what your daily caloric requirements are by using an online calculator, such as
http://manytools.org/handy/bmr-calculator

Once you have clearly in mind how many calories you should be consuming each day for fat loss, compare it to your numbers in the food journal. If you are over your required daily total, resolve to make the change tomorrow.

Chapter 7: The True Importance of Exercise

When we begin to exercise, our muscles have to work harder. This is the reaction to a process called aerobic respiration, and is how the body makes energy. To make energy, our body needs oxygen. To get it, the lungs begin to ventilate more quickly. The oxygen that comes into the body diffuses into the blood, which is pumped around the body by the heart. The heart beats faster to pump blood around the body more quickly. This provides the muscles with more oxygen. The muscles now have more oxygen to make more energy. This allows them to work harder.

Exercise where the heart and lungs work harder for a long period of time is known as aerobic training. Aerobic exercise has many benefits for the body, which is why it is recommended that we all do it for a minimum of thirty minutes each day.

Oxygen is carried around the body by red blood cells. When you train aerobically, your body makes more red blood cells. This makes your body a far more efficient transporter of oxygen. As a result, the arteries get bigger and more stretchy. This has the beneficial effect of lowering blood pressure because your heart doesn't have to work as hard to pump the blood around your body.

Aerobic exercise also causes more capillaries to form in the muscles, allowing oxygen to be delivered more quickly. When you exercise against a resistance, your body undergoes a hypertrophic effect, which enlarges the size of your muscles. As well as the skeletal muscles, the heart also gets stronger. Thicker muscles can contract more forcefully so they don't have to work as hard.

When you stop exercising, the time it takes for your heart rate to return to normal is called your recovery time. Recovery time decreases with exercise and improved fitness.

The diaphragm and intercostal muscles get stronger when you exercise. This makes your chest cavity larger when you breathe in. When you have a bigger chest cavity, more air can be taken in. This allows you to get more oxygen into your body. In addition, more capillaries grow around the air sacs in your lungs. These are called alveoli, and pass oxygen through the capillary walls and into the blood.

There are many physical benefits to regular physical exercise. It will improve your body shape, muscle tone and flexibility. It strengthens your bones, reduces the chance of illness, and increases your life expectancy. It will also increase your strength, endurance and muscle size.

In addition, exercise can give you an aim or goal, something to strive for. It can also be enjoyable, helping to reduce stress and tension levels. Exercise will help you to feel better about yourself, greatly enhancing your self-confidence.

Of course there are also social benefits to exercise. It can improve your teamwork and cooperation skills. It can also help you to meet new people, leading to new friendships.

Exercise for Fat Loss

Exercise, of course, is a very effective way to burn fat. Both aerobic and anaerobic exercise should be a part of your lifestyle as you combine diet and exercise to achieve the body that you deserve. What, though, are the most effective ways to work out to shed fat?

1) HIIT Training

High Intensity Interval Training is the fastest way to burn calories known to man. It involves short bursts of absolute maximum intensity cardio exercise with even shorter rest periods. 20-second sprints and 10-second rest periods are ideal. For maximum fat burning, both during and after the workout, do 8 cycles of this routine. The best exercises to choose from are stationery cycling, sprinting and rowing.

2) Weight Training

Many people fail to realize just how great a calorie burner weight training is. In fact, it's quite possible that weight training can burn more calories than cardio, especially if you include compound movements such as squats, lunges, presses, dead-lifts and rows. A huge bonus of weight training is that it provides a huge metabolic boost after the workout. In addition, when you increase your lean body mass, you'll be pushing your metabolic rate even higher. Train 2 days per week with high rep (12-20) sets of squats, lunges, dead-lifts, lat pull-downs, bench press and barbell curls.

Conclusion

Congratulations!

You now have the power to transform your body – and your life. Living the low carb lifestyle will allow you to take control of what you eat and how you feel. It will also give you the ultimate weight management tool.

In this book, we have shown you the why of low carb eating. We've also provided the how – with dozens of mouth-watering recipes to get you enthused, safe in the knowledge that sticking to your diet doesn't have to mean depriving yourself. We encourage you to create your own menu based on the delicious recipes that we've offered.

We've also provided guidance regarding the most effective forms of exercise to shed fat fast. We encourage you to do both cardio and resistance training regularly in order to achieve the body that you deserve.

You'll never regret choosing the low carb lifestyle.

Live it.

Embrace It.

Own It.

Your body will love you for it!